Three Filters and a Pump

Understanding Functions of the Heart

Lungs, Liver and Kidneys

To

Improve Your Health

By

Ayaz M. Samadani M.D.

First published date July 2005

ISBN 10: 0-9769065-0-3
ISBN 13: 978-0-976906-50-3

Publisher Farah Enterprises Ltd.

This book is printed on acid-free paper.
Printed in China.

Dedication

"I wish to share this knowledge with readers
to inform them of good health practices."

Acknowledgement

I wish to thank my family for their support and tolerance. I have taken their valuable time to get my thoughts together to put those thoughts into this book.

My gratitude and acknowledgement are due to my patients who inspired me to write this book. I have tried to answer in simple words their often-repeated questions.

I would like to express my gratitude to John Patterson, for his valuable advice and guidance in the writing of this book.

Table of Contents

TABLE OF CONTENTS   IX

THE PUMP   2

LAYERS OF THE HEART   8

ELECTRICAL IMPULSES   11

CARDIAC CYCLE   14

BLOOD FLOW THROUGH THE HEART   16

ARTERIAL BLOOD SUPPLY OF THE
HEART   17

UNDERSTANDING
ELECTROCARDIOGRAM   18

NORMAL ELECTROCARDIOGRAM   19

ELECTROCARDIOGRAM SHOWING
EXTRA VENTRICULAR CONTRACTION   20

DISEASES OF THE HEART   21

CORONARY ARTERY DISEASE AND HEART ATTACKS   22

NORMAL CORONARY LUMEN   22

WHAT IS A HEART ATTACK?   25

HEART ATTACK WARNING SIGNS   30

SIX KEY STEPS TO REDUCE HEART ATTACK RISK   31

CONTROL HIGH BLOOD PRESSURE   38

BLOOD PRESSURE APPARATUS   39

MONITOR   42

DIET THAT MAY HELP TO PREVENT HIGH BLOOD PRESSURE   44

PORTABLE BLOOD PRESSURE APPARATUS   47

MEDICATION   48

REDUCE HIGH BLOOD CHOLESTEROL   51

AIM FOR A HEALTHY WEIGHT 54

KEY RECOMMENDATIONS 57

HEART CATHETERIZATION 61

TWO STENTS ARE IN PLACE IN THE CORONARY ARTERY 62

STROKE 63

TYPES OF STROKES 64

TRANSIENT ISCHEMIC ATTACK (TIA) OR "MINI-STROKE." 65

LIVER 72

DISEASES OF THE LIVER 74

SOME OF THE SYMPTOMS MAY INCLUDE 78

DIAGNOSIS 78

ARE YOU AT RISK FOR HEPATITIS C? 79

LUNGS 82

STRUCTURE AND FUNCTION   84

LUNG AILMENTS MAY BE PRESENT AS   90

DISEASES OF THE LUNGS   91

KIDNEYS   98

BLOOD SUPPLY OF THE KIDNEY   98

STRUCTURE AND FUNCTION   99

URINE PRODUCTION   101

COMMON PROBLEMS AND COMPLICATIONS   102

BLOOD IN THE URINE   102

URINARY TRACT INFECTION   102

TEST   102

RULE OF THREE   107

LIFESTYLE CHANGES   108

Preface

From the creation of human beings to the present, no changes have occurred in the fundamental structure and composition of human body. With advancing age, however, certain changes do occur in the body. The heart, the most important organ next to the brain, starts its work in the first 6 weeks of gestation. The liver, lungs and kidneys depend on the function of the heart to get their blood supply. To understand these essential organs, one must understand the structure, anatomy and functions, and ailments of the organs.

This book explains the interdependency of these organs and their function. Understanding their interdependency should make it easier to understand the diseases of these organs and thus their treatment. Heart disease is the leading cause of death followed by strokes in third place. The national average for deaths due to cardiovascular disease is 336.6 per 100,000 populations. Cardiovascular disease, in-spite of improvement in medical care, remains the number one killer in the world. To prevent unnecessary early deaths, one must make changes in one's lifestyle. Now proven lifestyle changes can improve the outcome.

Early recognition of a disease and proper treatment will help the longevity of the patient.

Sensible eating and foods that include proper ingredients of essential nutrients is a must. Along with eating a routine exercise and activity program may help reduce the risk factors for developing multi organ disorders. Proper recognition of symptoms is a key to early interference and better outcome. After reading this book, the reader will have a clear concept how the heart, the liver, the lungs and the kidneys function. Common symptoms of disorders in these organs are described in an easy to understand manner. If we understand these organs it would become easier to get help at an early stage of disorder of these organs.

Introduction

Three Filters and a Pump

I have been a physician for over four decades and have practiced on three continents. I have dealt with all kinds of illnesses and emergencies. I have assisted in countless births and witnessed many people dying. I have also attended people struggling with their complicated illnesses. One thing is very clear: the basic body structure and functions are the same for people regardless of their geographical location or language differences.

There are several functions of the human body that are under one's own control. Good habits that maintain these body functions are necessary for maintaining optimal health.

The main body parts are comprised of four essential organs that I would like to focus on. The three filters described here are the liver, the lungs, and the kidneys, and the pump is the heart. Once these human organs are taken care of properly, good health and longevity should follow. In this book difficult medical terminology has been avoided as far as possible and simple, easy to understand language has been used.

This book describes the function, the structure, the most common malfunctions, the risk factors, the presentation of symptoms and the preventive measures so that one may understand the working mechanism of these organs. It is necessary to understand the components of the body and to see how they work in harmony. Once the function is known, taking care of these organs and recognizing the illnesses of these organs (malfunction) become easy to understand as well.

Ayaz M. Samadani M.D.

Three Filters and a Pump

Understanding Functions of the Heart
Lungs, Liver and Kidneys
To
Improve Your Health

The Pump

The Musculo-Neurological pump weighs 11 ounces and pumps 4300 gallons of blood in 24 hours without any rest or shutdown. All of the blood in the body passes through the heart in one minute.

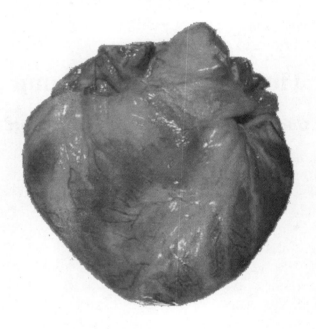

Human Heart

Heart

Structure and Function

The heart is a part of the cardiovascular system and its function is to supply the whole body with blood. It pumps about 4300 gallons of oxygen-rich blood throughout the body per day. All of our blood is pumped through our hearts about once every minute.

It is important to learn about the parts of the heart and to take care of this impressive organ, which enables the circulatory system to function. It is a muscular organ that weighs about 11 ounces and is shaped like an oval ball. It is located in the middle of the chest behind the breastbone, between the lungs. The heart rests in a fluid-filled sac called the pericardial cavity, which is surrounded by the ribcage. The diaphragm, a layer of muscle, lies below the heart. As a result, the heart is well protected. The heart contains several vessels, called veins and arteries, which carry blood in and out of the heart.

The heart is divided into two halves that are divided further into two chambers. A wall, called the septum, separates the right and left sides of the heart. These four chambers are called the right and the left ventricles and the right and the left atria.

3

The atria are the top two chambers that receive blood from the body or lungs. The ventricles are the bottom two chambers and they deliver blood to the body.

The left side of the heart pumps oxygenated blood through the aorta to the body.

The right side of the heart receives blood from the body and pumps it to the lungs for oxygenation.

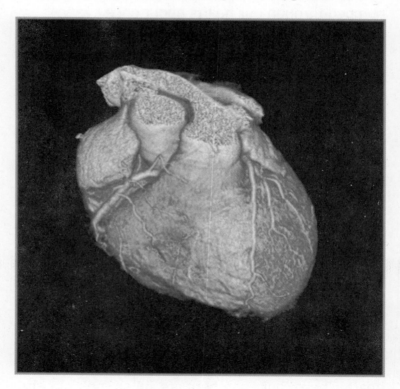

The right ventricle pumps blood to the lungs to pick up oxygen and the left ventricle, the strongest chamber, pumps blood to the head and the rest of the body.

The heart also contains valves, called atrioventricular valves and semilunar valves. Valves are flap-like structures that allow blood to flow in one direction and to prevent the backflow of blood.

Atrioventriuclar valves connect each atrium to the ventricle below it. The mitral valve connects the left atrium with the left ventricle and it prevents the backflow of blood as it is pumped between the left atrium and the left ventricle. The tricuspid valve connects the right atrium with the right ventricle and serves the same function as the mitral valve. Semilunar valves are located between the aorta and the left ventricle and the pulmonary artery and the right ventricle. They are appropriately called, the aortic valve and the pulmonary valve. The sounds that we hear the heart make, or the heart beat, are the sounds made when the heart valves close.

Blood is pumped away from the heart by the arteries and returned to the heart through the veins. The aorta, the pulmonary vessels and the vena cava are the main blood vessels. The aorta is the main artery of the body that delivers oxygenated blood to the body. It begins at the upper part of the left ventricle, where it is about 3 centimeters in diameter, and then it arches down and extends to the abdomen, where it branches off into two smaller arteries.

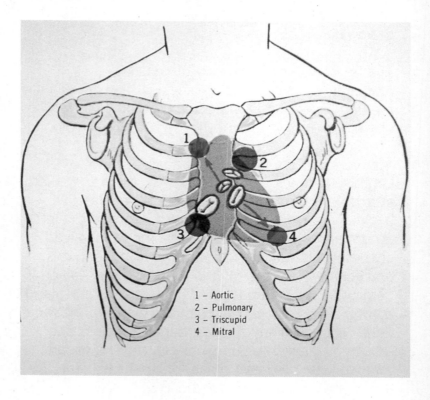

1 – Aortic
2 – Pulmonary
3 – Triscupid
4 – Mitral

The vena cavas are the two largest veins in the body. They are classified as the superior vena cava and the inferior vena cava. They carry de-oxygenated blood from various regions of the body to the right atrium.

The superior vena cava is responsible for bringing de-oxygenated blood from the head, neck and chest regions to the right atrium and the inferior vena cava brings de-oxygenated blood from the lower body regions to the right atrium.

The pulmonary artery extends from the right ventricle to the lungs and carries de-oxygenated blood between the right ventricle and lungs. The pulmonary vein extends from the left atrium to the lungs and carries oxygenated blood from the lungs to the left atrium.

Aorta
Left Atrium
Right Atrium
Left Ventricle
Right Ventricle

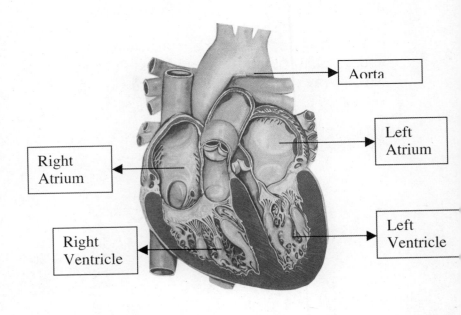

Four Chambers of the Heart

Layers of the Heart

The wall of the heart has three layers: the epicardium, the myocardium and the endocardium. The epicardium, also known as the pericardium, is the outer layer of the wall of the heart and provides a layer of protection for the heart. The myocardium, the middle layer, is composed of cardiac muscles, which allow the heart to contract in order to pump blood to and from the heart. The inner layer of the heart wall, the endocardium, lines the inner cavities of the heart and covers the heart valves. The endocardium contains nerves called Purkinje fibers, which relay cardiac impulses that cause the ventricles to contract.

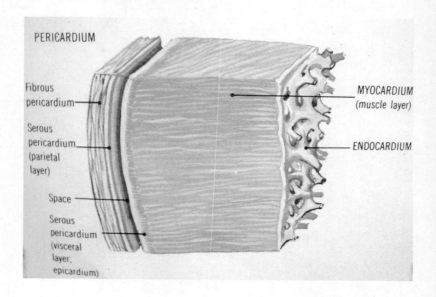

PERICARDIUM

Fibrous pericardium

Serous pericardium (parietal layer)

Space

Serous pericardium (visceral layer; epicardium)

MYOCARDIUM (muscle layer)

ENDOCARDIUM

A human being's heart is about the size of a fist. The average size and weight of the heart varies depending on age and sex. As the body develops, the heart grows at the same rate as the body. However, in the womb, that ratio is not the same.

The heart begins to develop between the second and sixth week of pregnancy. The ratio between the size of the heart and the size of the body is nine times greater in the fetus than in the infant. During the first few weeks after conception, the heart occupies most of the midsection. During the first few weeks of gestation, the heart is located high in the midsection. In time, it moves down to its position in the chest.

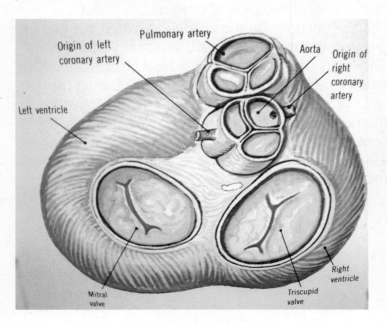

9

The four-chambered heart structure distinguishes the human heart, but the fetal heart must go through several phases to develop into that familiar shape. At first, the heart is just a tube. It grows so fast that it needs more space, so it bends and twists back, forming the familiar shape. During the next phase, the two atria are partly separate but there is just one big ventricle.

The next phase begins when the two atria are completely separate and the ventricles are just beginning to separate. Finally, the ventricles separate completely and the heart is developed.

The heart needs oxygen to grow, develop properly and stay healthy. Lack of oxygen can affect the heart's function. During childhood, when the body is growing the most, the heart needs more oxygen. The heart pumps oxygen-rich blood fastest during infancy, about 120 beats per minute. But as the child grows, and does not need as much oxygen, the heart rate slows. A nine-year-old child's heart beats about 90 times per minute compared to an 18-year-old, whose heart beats about 70 beats per minute.

Electrical Impulses

Cardiac conduction is the rate at which the heart conducts electrical impulses. These electrical impulses are caused by nodes. A node is a special type of tissue that acts like a muscle and a nerve. When nodal tissue contracts, like muscle tissue, it generates nerve impulses, like nervous tissue, that travel throughout the heart wall. Cardiac muscles, like those located in the myocardium, contract spontaneously.

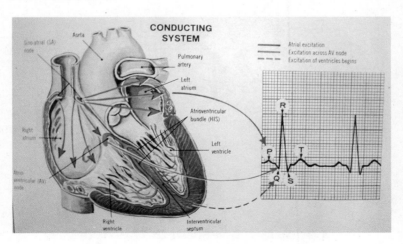

11

The conduction system of the heart. Sino-atrial node (SAN), Atrio-ventricular node (AVN) Right bundle (RB), Left bundle (LB)

The sinoatrial node, a section of nodal tissue located in the upper wall of the right atrium, controls these contractions and sets the rate of the contractions. It is also called the pacemaker of the heart. The sinoatrial node controls contractions by spontaneously contracting and generating nerve impulses that travel throughout the heart wall, causing both atria to contract.

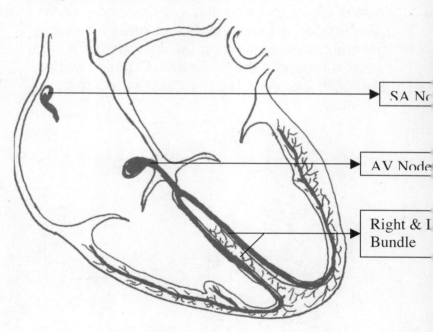

SA No

AV Node

Right & I
Bundle

Conduction System of the Heart

The atrioventricular node is located near the bottom of the right atrium. A tenth of a second delay occurs when the impulses reach the atrioventricular node, which allows the atria to contract and empty the blood that is in them. After the atrioventricular node, the impulses reach the atrioventricular bundle, fibers that are located within the septum of the heart.

The atroiventricular bundle splits into two more bundles of fibers, which carry the impulses down the center of the heart to the right and left ventricles. The fibers then branch into the Purkinje fibers at the base of the heart that cause the muscle fibers in the ventricles to contract.

Cardiac Cycle

The cardiac cycle is the sequence of events that occurs when the heart beats. There are two phases of this cycle called diastole (relaxed) and systole (contracted). These correspond to the numbers by which you determine how fast your heart is beating.

Diastole- Relaxed Phase

The diastole phase is divided into three parts: early diastole, mid diastole and late diastole. During the early diastole phase, the ventricles relax; semilunar valves close, atrioventricular valves open and the ventricles fill with blood. During the mid diastole phase, the atria and ventricles are both relaxed, the semilunar valves are closed and the atrioventricular valves are open and the ventricles continue to fill with blood. Finally, during the late diastole phase, the sinoatrial node contracts, the atria contract, the ventricles fill with more blood and the contraction reaches the atrioventricular node. After the diastole phase, the contraction passes from the atrioventricular node to the Purkinje fibers and ventricular cells during the systole phase.

Systole- Contraction Phase

During the systole phase, the ventricles contract, the atrioventricular valves close, the semilunar valves open, and blood is pumped from the ventricles to the arteries. The pulmonary valve keeps the blood from flowing back into the right ventricle. The pulmonary artery then carries the blood to the lungs where the blood picks up oxygen and is then returned to the left atrium by the pulmonary veins. Similarly the mitral valve keeps the blood from flowing back into the left ventricle. The aorta then carries the oxygenated blood to the brain and rest of the body.

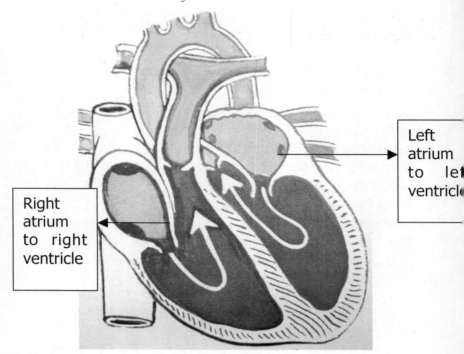

Right atrium to right ventricle

Left atrium to left ventricle

Blood Flow through the Heart

Coronary Arteries

Although the heart contains blood and supplies every cell in the body with oxygenated blood, it does not get any nourishment from the blood inside it. The function of the coronary arteries is to deliver blood to nourish the heart muscle. The coronary arteries branch off from the aorta into the left coronary artery and the right coronary artery. The left coronary artery delivers blood to the walls of the ventricles and the left atrium and right coronary artery delivers blood to the walls of the ventricles and right atrium. Any blockage in these arteries results in damage to that particular part of the heart resulting in a heart attack.

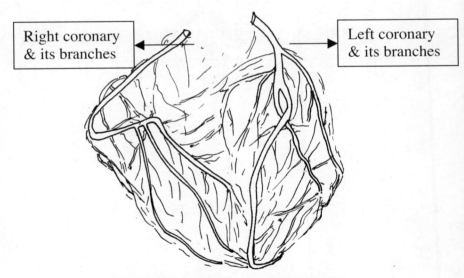

Right coronary & its branches

Left coronary & its branches

Arterial Blood Supply of the Heart

Understanding Electrocardiogram

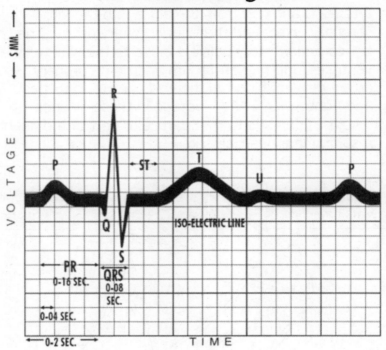

The Normal electrocardiogram tracing

SA node generates an electrical impulse that is shown on the cardiogram by PQ and AV node

generates an electrical impulse that is shown by
QRS interval.

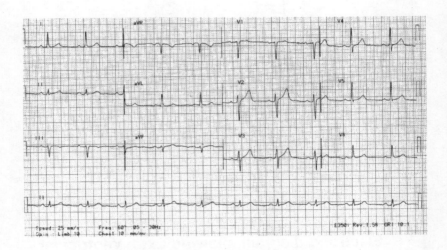

Normal Electrocardiogram

When these nodes are generating impulses
independently then irregular heart beats result as
shown by this following electrocardiogram (EKG).
These extra beats are called PACs (premature atrial
contractions) or PVCs (premature ventricular
contractions) depending on their source of origin.

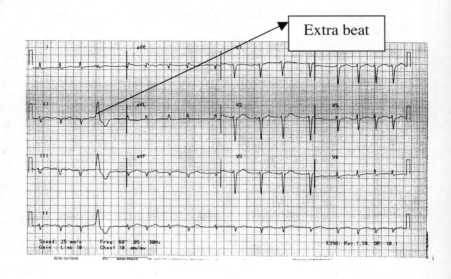

Extra beat

Electrocardiogram showing Extra Ventricular Contraction

Extra beats need to be treated under certain conditions as blood may not be pumped properly if the heart is beating rapidly without getting time to refill the cavities by blood. Irregular heart beat may result from lack of blood supply or heart muscle damage.

Diseases of the Heart

Now that you know how your pump functions, let's discuss what can go wrong with the heart if it is not properly taken care of. Diseases affecting the heart are very serious and lethal. In fact, heart and blood vessel disease is the number one killer in the nation and a stroke is the number three killer. Heart attacks and chest pain cause about half of heart and blood vessel disease-related deaths. In the United States alone about 250,000 people die every year even before they get to the hospital. Knowledge about these diseases, how to prevent them and what to do in case you suffer from them, may save your life.

Heart Failure

Pump failure or heart failure occurs when there is increased resistance to outflow or weakness in the heart muscle. This creates a back load and fluid build up in the lungs causing shortness of breath and swelling of the ankles. Retention of fluid in the body results in lung congestion and fluid in the lungs thus decreasing the capacity of air in the lungs. This results in shortness of breath, difficulty in walking due to shortness of breath, weight gain due to fluid retention, lack of energy and inability to lie flat in bed. Most of these patients spend their night sitting or sleeping in a reclining chair. Chest x-rays and echocardiograms help in making the final diagnosis. There are a number of medicines that help treat and control heart failure.

Coronary Artery Disease and Heart Attacks

A heart attack occurs when there is a blockage in one of the coronary arteries, which supply blood to the heart. Blood supply to the heart muscle, the myocardium, is cut off. If the blood supply is cut off for too long, more than just a few minutes, it can cause severe, permanent damage to the heart muscle, which can disable or kill the victim. Coronary artery disease, also called atherosclerosis, is the most common cause of a heart attack. Coronary artery disease is caused when fatty matter, called plaque, builds up in the coronary arteries. Deposits of cholesterol, cellular waste products, calcium and other substances in the coronary artery also cause the build up. The artery is damaged and roughened as it increasingly narrows due to the accumulation of plaque.

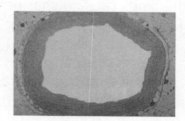

Normal coronary lumen

The narrowing of the artery prevents blood from flowing to the heart. Plaque can also rupture and cause a blood clot that completely blocks blood flow to the heart. Another factor of coronary heart disease is the accumulation of platelets, cells that cause blood to clot. Diseased arteries can also spasm, which further narrows the artery and blocks blood flow to the heart.

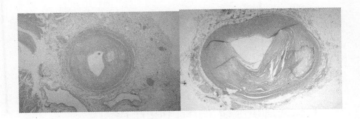

Occluded coronary lumen

Although some heart attacks are sudden, most begin slowly and happen before the victim knows what is happening. Often, he or she waits too long to get help and the heart suffers from permanent damage. Knowing the early warning signs of a heart attack can help you act quickly if you think you are having a heart attack.

Common Symptoms and History Related with Heart Attacks

- Exposure to emotional stress, extreme heat or cold.
- Consuming heavy meals.
- Alcohol and cigarette smoking.
- Dull aching or burning in chest area.
- Palpitations or rapid heart beats.
- Fast heart rate or skipped heart beats.
- Pressure, squeezing or fullness in the chest or upper part of the pit of the stomach.
- Pain or discomfort in one or both arms, back, neck, jaw or stomach.
- Shortness of breath.
- Cold sweat.
- Nausea.
- Lightheadedness.
- Dizziness.

What is a Heart Attack?

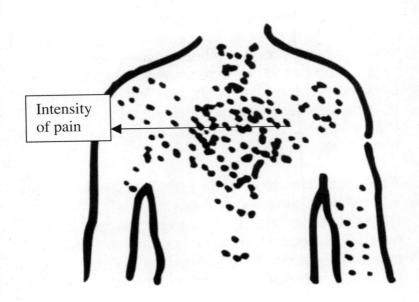

Intensity of pain

Severity of pain distribution in a heart attack
Early warning signs of a heart attack include recurring chest pressure or discomfort. This may feel like pressure, squeezing or fullness in the chest or upper part of the pit of the stomach. This may also be accompanied by pain or discomfort in one or both arms, back, neck, jaw or stomach. One might

also experience shortness of breath, cold sweat, nausea or lightheadedness. Angina pectoris is a similar type of chest pain or pressure in the heart, and is usually a sign that the heart is not receiving enough oxygen. Angina occurs when the heart's need for oxygen exceeds the amount of oxygen available from the blood fed to the heart through the coronary arteries. It is a common symptom of coronary artery disease, but can also be caused by emotional stress, extreme heat or cold, heavy meals, alcohol and cigarette smoking. In addition to pain and pressure, one might also feel dull aching or burning, palpitations, which feel like a fluttering in the chest, an accelerated heart rate or skipped heart beats.

All of these symptoms occur when the coronary arteries have narrowed so much that they can no longer supply enough blood, carrying oxygen, to the heart. The medical term for this condition is called ischemia. Angina is a sign of coronary artery disease, which can lead to a heart attack.

A heart attack can also occur without any warning symptoms at all. Also, angina will feel different from indigestion or heartburn. These occur after eating a heavy or spicy meal. Gallbladder disease or a stomach ulcer can also cause a similar pain.

It is important to note that an episode of angina is not a heart attack; angina means that the heart is not receiving enough oxygen, temporarily. There are certain differences between angina and a heart attack. When one suffers from angina, the blood supply to the heart is blocked temporarily and the symptoms last for a short period of time. The symptoms are relieved with rest and/or medications.

Angina does not cause permanent damage to the heart muscle. In the case of a heart attack blood supply to the heart is blocked for an extended period of time, the symptoms last longer, usually 30 minutes, the symptoms persist, even with rest or medication, and may result in permanent damage to the heart muscle. When one suffer from a stable pattern of angina it does not mean that a heart attack is about to occur. However, if there is a change in the angina pattern, the risk of heart attack is much higher.

Furthermore, people who suffer from angina are at a greater risk of a heart attack.

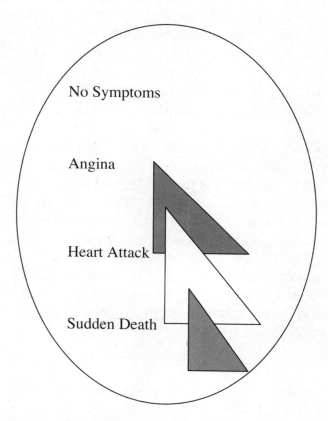

The majorities with coronary artery disease do not show any symptoms. As the narrowing of the lumen continues for many years, diminished blood supply, angina, heart attack and sudden death may result.

Risk Factors

Some factors leading to a heart attack cannot be controlled, such as a family history of cardiovascular disease. These people are at a higher risk for coronary artery disease. Males are at a higher risk than females, but that doesn't mean that women don't have to be careful. After menopause women have the same risk as men of their age group. However, you can control and change many factors in order to have a healthier lifestyle and prevent certain cardiovascular diseases. These are called risk factors and they include: smoking cigarettes, high cholesterol level, high blood pressure, obesity, lack of physical activity and weight gain. Having more than one of these risk factors increases the chances of having a heart attack.

Heart Attack Warning Signs

A heart attack is a frightening event, and you probably don't want to think about it. But, if you learn the signs of a heart attack and what steps to take, you can save a life—maybe your own.
What are the signs of a heart attack? Many people think a heart attack is sudden and intense, like a "movie" heart attack, where a person clutches his or her chest and falls over.
The truth is that many heart attacks start slowly, as a mild pain or discomfort. If you feel such a symptom, you may not be sure what's wrong. Your symptoms may even come and go. Even those who have had a heart attack may not recognize their symptoms, because the next attack can have entirely different ones.

It's vital that everyone learn the warning signs of a heart attack. These are:

Chest discomfort. Most heart attacks involve discomfort in the center of the chest that lasts for more than a few minutes, or goes away and comes back. The discomfort can feel like uncomfortable pressure, squeezing, fullness, or pain.

Discomfort in other areas of the upper body. The discomfort can include pain or discomfort in one or both arms, the back, neck, jaw, or stomach.

Shortness of breath. Often comes along with chest discomfort. But it also can occur before chest discomfort.

Other symptoms. May include breaking out in a cold sweat, nausea, or light-headedness.
Source: NIH Library

Learn the signs—but also remember: Even if you're not sure it's a heart attack, you should still have it checked out. Fast action can save lives-maybe your own.

Six Key Steps to Reduce Heart Attack Risk

Taking these steps will reduce your risk of having a heart attack:

- Stop smoking
- Lower high blood pressure
- Reduce high blood cholesterol
- Aim for a healthy weight
- Be physically active each day
- Manage diabetes

Stop Smoking Cigarettes

Cigarette smoking greatly increases the risk of fatal and nonfatal heart attacks in both men and women. It also increases the risk of a second heart attack among survivors. Women who smoke and use oral contraceptives have an even greater risk. The good news is that quitting smoking greatly reduces the risk of heart attack. One year after quitting, the risk drops to about one-half that of current smokers and gradually returns to normal in persons without heart disease. Even among persons with heart disease, the risk also drops sharply one year after quitting smoking and it continues to decline over time but the risk does not return to normal.

The U.S. Food and Drug Administration have approved five medications to help you stop smoking and lessen the urge to smoke. They are:

- Bupropion SR - available by prescription

- Nicotine gum - available over-the-counter

- Nicotine inhaler - available by prescription

- Nicotine nasal spray - available by prescription

- Nicotine patch - available by prescription and over-the-counter

All of these medicines will more or less double your chances of quitting and quitting for good.

Preventable Death under Your Control

- Stop smoking cigarettes.
- Avoid second hand smoke.

Cigarette Smoking

Smoking is the leading risk factor in peripheral vascular disease, which restricts blood flow to the legs and lower part of the body. Furthermore, peripheral vascular disease almost exclusively affects smokers and can result in gangrene and amputation of the leg. Smokers' chances of having a heart attack are double those of non-smokers. Furthermore, smokers who have a heart attack are more likely to die than non-smokers who have a heart attack. This is because tobacco contains the addictive ingredient nicotine and carbon monoxide, which reduce the amount of oxygen that the heart receives.

The nicotine creates a strong craving for another cigarette, making it very difficult to quit smoking. Nicotine is a stimulant to the brain and nervous system. It causes the heart to beat faster and blood pressure to rise. It also contributes to the build up of plaque on blood vessel walls. Another risk associated with smoking is that it can cause blood clots and reduce HDL, which is good cholesterol. With all of these increased risks due to smoking, the best thing for smokers to do is quit right away. Smoking damages blood vessel walls, but your risk is greatly reduced as soon as you stop smoking.

If you don't smoke, don't start. Moreover, constant exposure to secondhand smoke is also damaging to the non-smoker, so avoid other people's smoke even if you don't smoke.

- Nicotine is addictive.
- One in five Americans smokes cigarettes.
- 47 million individuals in U.S. smoke.
- Smokers on the average cut 14 years of their life.

Smoking Cessation Programs Improve Survival

New findings from the Lung Health Study (LHS) show that intensive smoking cessation programs can significantly improve long-term survival among smokers. LHS is a landmark study that differs from many other studies of cigarette smoking in that it was a randomized, controlled clinical trial -- considered the gold standard in determining cause and effect; furthermore, the size and duration of LHS enabled it to measure more accurately the risks associated with smoking than other clinical trials.

LHS followed nearly 5,900 middle-aged smokers who had mild to moderately abnormal lung function but were otherwise healthy when they enrolled in the study. Participants were assigned to either a 10-week intensive smoking cessation program or to usual care (no intervention).

The intervention program included behavior modification and use of nicotine gum, with a continuing five-year maintenance program to minimize relapse. After five years, approximately 22 percent of the participants in the smoking cessation program were sustained quitters, with nearly 90 percent of them continuing their success after 11 years. About 5 percent of those who did not receive the intervention were sustained quitters after five years. After an average of 14.5 years, the death rate among those in the smoking cessation program was about 15 percent lower compared to those who received the usual care. The results are published in the Annals of Internal Medicine.

Cigarette Smoking or Second Hand Smoke

- Increases risk of coronary heart disease.
- Increases risk of heart attack.
- Increases risk of Stroke.
- Lowers HDL, good cholesterol.
- Interferes with oxygen in the blood.
- Increases respiratory problems.
- Is the leading cause of death from lung cancer.
- Increases incidence of spontaneous pneumothorax.

Control High Blood Pressure

High blood pressure makes the heart work harder. It increases the risk of developing heart disease, as well as kidney disease and stroke. High blood pressure in medical terms is called hypertension. It usually has no symptoms. Once developed, it typically lasts a lifetime.

Blood pressure is recorded as two numbers–the systolic pressure (as the heart beats) over the diastolic pressure (as the heart relaxes). For example, a measurement would be written as 120/80 mm Hg (millimeters of mercury).

Normal blood pressure is less than 130 mm Hg systolic and less than 85 mm Hg diastolic. An optimal blood pressure is less than 120 mm Hg systolic and less than 80 mm Hg diastolic. A consistent blood pressure reading of 140/90 mm Hg or higher is considered high blood pressure. If the systolic and diastolic pressures fall into different categories, the higher category is used to classify blood pressure status.

Blood Pressure Apparatus

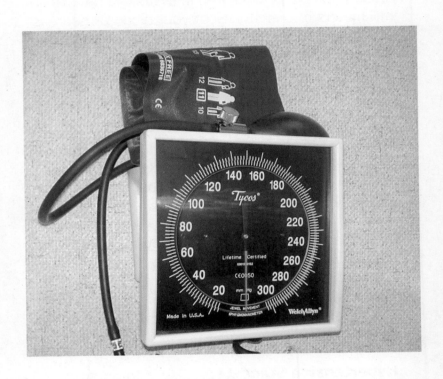

Screening for High Blood Pressure

Blood pressure is measured in systolic and diastolic millimeters of mercury. So if your blood pressure is 120/80, it means that your systolic blood pressure is 120 and your diastolic pressure is 80. Blood pressure is high if two readings 1-2 weeks apart measures 140/90 or above.

Pre-hypertension:
This is the stage where you are at risk of developing high blood pressure. This is the time that lifestyle changes may help to keep your blood pressure from getting worse.

More than120-139 Systolic and >80-89 Diastolic mmHg.

Hypertension Stage 1:
More than 140-159 Systolic and 90-99 Diastolic mmHg.

Hypertension Stage 11:
More than 160 Systolic and 100 Diastolic mmHg.

Keep your Blood Pressure at 120/80 mmHg.

There are two forces that create blood pressure. The heart creates one as it pumps blood into the arteries and through the circulatory system. The other is the force of the arteries as they resist the blood flow. High blood pressure is caused by constricted arterioles, which are smaller arteries. Blood is pumped through the arteries in arterioles by the heart. When the arterioles contract or expand, it alters the resistance to the blood flow. This, in turn, affects the amount of blood flow and the blood pressure. When the arterioles contract, there is more resistance to blood flow because there is a smaller space for the blood to pass through. This increases blood pressure. Expansion of the arterioles has the opposite affect on blood flow and blood pressure.

Monitor

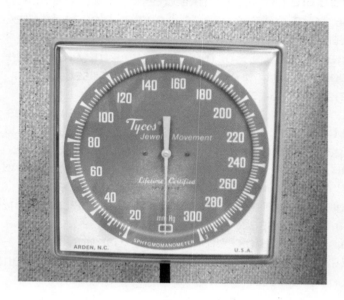

High blood pressure is called the "silent killer" because many people have it for years without ever knowing about it. High blood pressure usually does not have any symptoms, so the only way to diagnose it is to have your blood pressure checked. In most cases, 90-95%, it is unknown what causes high blood pressure. These cases are called essential hypertension and can be influenced by atherosclerosis, thickening of the artery wall and constricted arteries.

The remaining 5-10% of cases of high blood pressure are caused by secondary hypertension. Causes of secondary hypertension include a kidney abnormality, a tumor in the adrenal gland or a congenital defect of the aorta. Blood pressure usually returns to normal when these causes are treated.

Certain diet and lifestyle changes may help alleviate high blood pressure such as maintaining a diet that is rich in calcium, potassium, magnesium and protein and low in total fat, saturated fat, cholesterol and sodium. Losing weight, lowering alcohol intake and exercising regularly can also lower blood pressure. If simple diet and lifestyle changes do not help, there are also medications that people can take to help lower blood pressure.

How do you know that your blood pressure is high?

Most of the time high blood pressure does not cause any symptoms and people do not know they have high blood pressure. Usually they find out that blood pressure is elevated during a routine medical visit.

Symptoms most likely to be associated with high blood pressure are:

- Headache.
- Chest pain or tightness in the chest.
- Feeling lightheaded or dizzy.
- Shortness of breath.
- Rapid heart beat or pulse.
- Feeling weak.
- Problems with vision or hearing.
- Impotence.

Diet that may help to prevent high blood pressure

- Dietary fish and fish oil.
- Low sodium, low chloride diet.
- Adequate calcium intake.
- Fiber or indigestible carbohydrates.
- Consuming un-saturated fats.
- Proper magnesium intake.

Instructions on how to use the blood pressure equipment

You should become familiar with the blood pressure equipment.

Cuff:

Place the cuff above the elbow with the flat of the diaphragm of the bell against the skin or over one thin layer of clothing on the inside of the arm at the bend of the elbow. Tighten the cuff in place by using velcro. Make a smooth wrap around the upper arm.

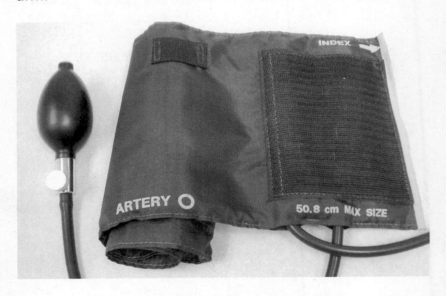

Stethoscope:
Place the earpiece tips in the ears. Tips should be facing slightly out and downwards.
Bulb:
Hold the rubber bulb in your dominant hand. Close the valve by turning away from you with the index finger and the thumb. Squeeze the bulb several times. Watch the needle on the dial of the monitor. You can use one hand to squeeze the bulb and the other hand to hold the monitor. You can attach the monitor to the upper end of the wrapped cuff. If the cuff does not hold due to loose velcro or large size of the arm then use a larger cuff.

Squeezing the bulb will create pressure in the cuff that will raise numbers on the gauge. Squeeze the bulb
repeatedly until needle on the gauge reaches around 180 mark. Then slowly turn the valve towards you with your thumb and index finger.

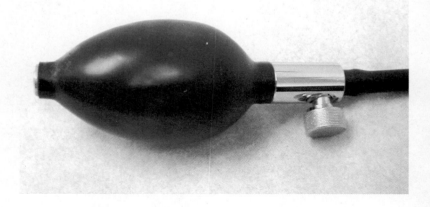

As the pressure is released in the cuff you should be able to hear a dub-dub sound. This indicates the top pressure. Remember this number on which you heard the sound first. Continue releasing the pressure. When the sound disappears note the number at which the needle is pointing. This is your lower blood pressure. If you get constant high reading then consult your health care provider.

Portable Blood Pressure Apparatus

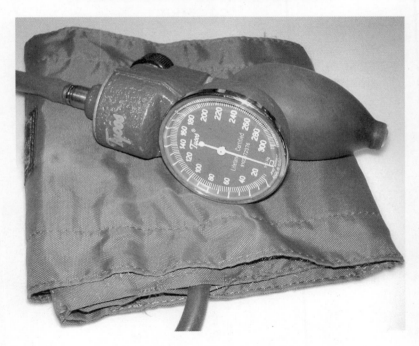

Blood Pressure Checking Intervals

Normal   120/80 mmHg, recheck in 1 years
High Normal 140/89 mmHg, recheck in 6 months
Hypertension over 140/90 mmHg, see a physician

Common Treatment of High Blood Pressure.

Lifestyle modification is necessary by controlling weight, stopping smoking cigarettes, reducing alcohol intake and exercising routinely.

Medication

Diuretics or water pills are most commonly used alone or with other medication to control high blood pressure. Add on medication is B-blocker or ACE (Angiotensin converting enzyme inhibitor) inhibitors. Patients who have coronary heart disease will need beta blocker or ACE inhibitor. Patients with heart failure benefit from use of ACE inhibitor or Angiotensin receptor blocker (ARB). In heart attack cases B-blocker and ACE-I are commonly used. In diabetes Mellitus ACE-I or ARB is first agent and second agent is B-blocker. African American patients with high blood pressure have better response to diuretic or ACE-I.

Diuretic
Chlorthalidone
Hydrochlorothiazide (Hydrodiuril)
Bumetanide (Bumex)
Furosemide (Lasix)
Triamterene (Diazide, Dyrenium)

B-blocker
Acebutol (Sectral)
Atenolol (Tenormin)
Bisoprolol (Ziac)
Metoprolol (Lopressor, Toprol XL)
Nadolol (Corgard)
Pindolol
Propranolol (Inderal, InnoPran XL)
Timolol (Blocadren)

Ace inhibitor
Benzepril (Lotensin)
Captopril (Capoten)
Enalapril (Vasotec)
Lisinopril (Prinivil, Zestril)
Quinapril (Accupril)
Ramipril (Altace)
Trandolapril (Mavik, Tarka)

A & B-blocker
Labetalol (Normodyne, Trandate)
Carvedilol (Coreg)

ARB
Losartan (Cozaar, Hyzaar)
Valsartan (Diovan, -HCT)

Calcium channel blocker
Verapamil (Calan,-SR, Covera HS, Isoptin SR,
Verelan,-PM, Tarka)
Diltiazem (Cardizem LA-CD-SR-XR, Tiazac)

Dihydropyridine calcium channel blocker
Felodipine (Plendil, Lexxel)
Amlodipine (Norvasc, Lotrel)
Isradipine (DynaCirc,-CR)
Nicardipine (Cardene,-SR)
Nifedipine (Adalat CC, Procardia XL)
Nisoldipine (Sular)

Goal of Therapy
Keep a reading near130/85mmHg or less.

Reduce High Blood Cholesterol

The level of cholesterol in the bloodstream greatly affects the risk of developing heart disease. The higher the level of blood cholesterol, the greater the risk for heart disease or heart attacks.

Why? When there is too much cholesterol (a fat-like substance) in the blood, it builds up in the walls of arteries. Over time, this buildup causes arteries to become narrowed, and blood flow to the heart is slowed or blocked. If the blood supply to a portion of the heart is completely cut off, a heart attack results.
Various factors affect cholesterol levels: diet, weight, physical activity, age and gender, and heredity.

High blood cholesterol itself does not cause symptoms. You may not know your blood cholesterol level is too high. So, it is important to have your cholesterol measured. Adults age 20 or older should have their cholesterol checked at least once every 5 years. It is best to have a blood test called a lipoprotein profile. This test measures total cholesterol, "good" and "bad" cholesterol, as well as triglycerides, another form of fat in the blood.

High cholesterol is treated with

- Lifestyle changes–a heart healthy eating plan
- Physical activity
- Loss of excess weight
- Medications that include Statins, Bile acid sequestrants, Nicotinic acid and Fibric acids

Cholesterol is a soft, fatty substance found in the body and all of its cells. Some cholesterol is good and necessary for bodily functions, such as building cell membranes, some hormones and other tissues, but other cholesterol is bad. There are two ways that people get cholesterol: the body produces it and it is also ingested in food. Cholesterol is carried through the body by lipoproteins, which are made by the liver. The liver produces about 1,000 mg per day and another 400-500 mg comes from foods.

Goals
Total Cholesterol   Goal <200
HDL (Good Cholesterol) Goal >40 Men   >50 Women
LDL (Bad Cholesterol) Goal <100
Triglycerides Goal <150

The body generally produces all of the cholesterol that it needs, so it is not necessary to get it from outside food sources. High cholesterol does not have any symptoms, so it is necessary to get it checked regularly. Cholesterol is measured in milligrams per deciliter of blood, which is abbreviated mg/dL.

There are two main types of cholesterol – Low-density lipoprotein (LDL), bad cholesterol, and high-density lipoprotein (HDL), good cholesterol. Carrying 60 to 80 percent of the body's cholesterol, LDL cholesterol is the main cholesterol carrier in the body. This cholesterol is used to build cells; what is not used to build cells is returned to the liver. When there is too much LDL cholesterol in the body, it can build up on the walls of the coronary arteries, leading to coronary artery disease. A healthy level of LDL cholesterol is less than 100 mg/dL. A LDL cholesterol level of 160 mg/dL is considered high and raises a person's risk of having a heart attack.

HDL cholesterol is good because high levels may protect against a heart attack by removing excess cholesterol from constricted arteries and carrying it back to liver, where it is then discharged from the body. Low HDL cholesterol level, lower than 40 mg/dL, increases one's risk of a heart attack and stroke.

It has been proven that women have higher HDL cholesterol levels than men because estrogen raises HDL cholesterol levels. This may explain why men are at greater risk for cardiovascular diseases.

Triglycerides are another type of fat in the body that put people at risk for heart disease. Triglycerides are actually the most common type of fat in the body and are carried together with HDL cholesterol and LDL cholesterol by lipoproteins.

Although normal triglyceride levels vary depending on age and sex, generally less than 150mg/dL is considered normal and 200 mg/dL is high. Age and/or weight gain tend to increase in triglyceride levels.

Aim for a Healthy Weight

A healthy weight is crucial for a long, healthy life. Being overweight or obese increases your risk of a heart attack. It increases your risk of developing high blood cholesterol, high blood pressure, and diabetes-each of which also increase your chance of having a heart attack. If you are overweight, even a small weight loss, just 10 percent of your current weight, will help to lower your risk of developing these diseases.

Two of the measures that assess whether or not a person is overweight are body mass index (BMI) and waist circumference. BMI is a measure of weight relative to height. Waist circumference measures abdominal fat. The risk for developing heart and other diseases increases with a waist measurement of more than 40 inches in men and more than 35 inches in women.

Body mass index (BMI) is measure of body fat based on height and weight that applies to both adult men and women.

BMI Categories:
Underweight = <18.5
Normal weight = 18.5-24.9
Overweight = 25-29.9
Obesity = BMI of 30 or greater

To be at their best, adults need to avoid gaining weight and many needs to lose weight. Losing weight and keeping it off depends on a change of lifestyle that combines sensible eating with regular physical activity, not a temporary effort to drop pounds quickly. If you need to lose excess weight, talk with your health care provider about developing an action plan, which includes a heart-healthy, low-calorie, nutritious eating plan and physical activity.

Obesity and physical inactivity are also risk factors for heart attacks. People who are overweight often have other health problems, such as high blood pressure and high cholesterol, which contribute to their risk. Even a small amount of weight loss can decrease one's risk of heart disease.

Therefore, it is important to stay physically active and maintain a healthy diet. Another risk factor is stress. People who have high stress and cannot control it often have health problems.

In 2005, 65% of adult Americans are overweight or obese, and 16% of American children are overweight. If you are overweight or obese, carrying this extra weight puts you at risk for developing many diseases.

Key Recommendations

(From the Expert Panel on the Identification, Evaluation, and Treatment of Overweight and Obesity in Adults-*NIH data*)

Weight loss to lower elevated blood pressure in overweight and obese persons with high blood pressure.

Weight loss to lower elevated levels of total cholesterol, LDL-cholesterol, and triglycerides, and to raise low levels of HDL-cholesterol in overweight and obese persons with dyslipidemia.

Weight loss to lower elevated blood glucose levels in overweight and obese persons with type 2 diabetes.

Use the BMI to assess overweight and obesity. Body weight alone can be used to follow weight loss, and to determine the effectiveness of therapy.

The BMI to classify overweight and obesity and to estimate relative risk of disease compared to normal weight.

The waist circumference should be used to assess abdominal fat content.

The initial goal of weight loss therapy should be to reduce body weight by about 10 percent from baseline.

Weight loss should be about 1 to 2 pounds per week for a period of 6 months, with the subsequent strategy based on the amount of weight lost.

Low calorie diets (LCD) for weight loss in overweight and obese persons. Reducing fat as part of an LCD is a practical way to reduce calories.

Reducing dietary fat alone without reducing calories is not sufficient for weight loss. However, reducing dietary fat, along with reducing dietary carbohydrates, can help reduce calories.

A diet that is individually planned to help create a deficit of 500 to 1,000 kcal/day should be an integral part of any program aimed at achieving a weight loss of 1 to 2 pounds per week.

Physical activity should be part of a comprehensive weight loss therapy and weight control program because it:

- Modestly contributes to weight loss in overweight and obese adults.
- May decrease abdominal fat.
- Increases cardio respiratory fitness.

- May help with maintenance of weight loss.

Initially, moderate levels of physical activity for 30 to 45 minutes, 3 to 5 days a week, should be encouraged. All adults should set a long-term goal to accumulate at least 30 minutes or more of moderate-intensity physical activity on most, and preferably all, days of the week.

The combination of a reduced calorie diet and increased physical activity is recommended since it produces weight loss that may also result in decreases in abdominal fat and increases in cardio respiratory fitness.

After successful weight loss, the likelihood of weight loss maintenance is enhanced by a program consisting of dietary therapy, physical activity, and behavior therapy, which should be continued indefinitely.

Drug therapy can also be used. However, drug safety and efficacy beyond 1 year of total treatment have not been established.

A weight maintenance program should be a priority after the initial 6 months of weight loss therapy.

Be Physically Active Each Day

Being physically active reduces the risk of heart-related problems, including heart attack. Physical activity can improve cholesterol levels, help control high blood pressure and diabetes, and manage weight. It also increases physical fitness, promotes psychological well-being and self-esteem, and reduces depression and anxiety.

Those who have already had a heart attack also benefit greatly from being physically active. Many hospitals have a cardiac (or heart) rehabilitation program. A health care provider can offer advice about a suitable program.

To protect your heart, you only need to do 30 minutes of a moderate-intensity activity on most and, preferably, all days of the week. If 30 minutes is too much at one time, you can break it up into periods of at least 10 minutes each.
If you have been inactive, you should start slowly to increase your physical activity.

If you have coronary heart disease, check with you health care provider before starting a physical activity program. This is especially important if you are over age 55, have been inactive, or have diabetes or another medical problem. Your health care provider can give you advice on how rigorous the exercise should be.

Heart Catheterization

To make a diagnosis of coronary artery disease a catheter is placed in the heart via blood vessels in the groin area. The progress of the catheter is watched on the screen under fluoroscopic examination. Once the tip of the catheter is in the coronary blood vessel a dye is injected and pictures taken. These pictures, still or a movie, show the narrow parts of the blood vessels.

In the same procedure a balloon or a stent may be placed in the narrow coronary blood vessels to open and keep open the narrow lumen. This procedure improves the blood supply to the heart muscle. Similarly a pace maker for heart block or a defibrillator is inserted to manage heart rate and to deliver a shock in case of ventricular fibrillation that may be fatal.

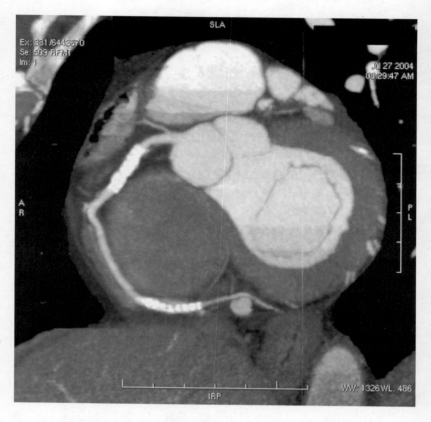

Two stents are in place in the coronary artery

Stroke

A stroke is another type of cardiovascular disease. A stroke, however, affects the blood vessels that supply blood to the brain. A stroke occurs when part of the brain does not get the oxygen it needs because of a blood clot or a rupture in an artery that supplies blood to the brain. Nerve cells in the area can't function without oxygen and die within minutes of blockage. Strokes often cause permanent damage to brain cells and the part of the body that they control.

Like a heart attack, certain risk factors affect one's chances of having a stroke. Many of them can be controlled, but others cannot. High blood pressure, diabetes mellitus, carotid artery disease, atrial fibrillation, smoking, blood disorders, sickle cell anemia, high cholesterol and obesity are all risk factors that contribute to strokes. Age, sex, heredity and a history of prior heart attack or stroke are factors that cannot be controlled. Additionally, women who smoke and use birth control pills may also be at risk.

Types of Strokes

There are two main types of strokes. They are those that are caused by a blockage and those that are caused by a ruptured blood vessel. These two types are further divided into two more types of stokes. Cerebral thrombosis and cerebral embolism are two types of strokes that are caused by a blood clot or other particle blocking the artery. This type of stroke accounts for 70-80 percent of all strokes. Cerebral and subarachnoid hemorrhages are caused by ruptured arteries and have a higher fatality rate than strokes caused by blocked arteries.

Cerebral thrombosis, which is the most common type of stroke, occurs when a blood clot forms and blocks blood flow in an artery that carries blood to the brain. As discussed above, blood clots form in arteries that suffer from atherosclerosis. This type of stroke occurs when blood pressure is low, at night or in the morning, and may follow a transient ischemic attack (TIA) or "mini-stroke."

Ayaz M. Samadani M.D.

Transient Ischemic Attack (TIA) or "Mini-Stroke."

A TIA feels like a stroke, but does not cause any permanent damage. A cerebral embolism is caused by a clot or particle that get stuck in the artery that brings blood to the brain and, thus, cuts off blood supply to the brain. The clot is usually formed elsewhere, like in the heart or lungs, and is then carried in the blood until it lodges in the artery feeding the brain.

The two types of stroke caused by a ruptured vessel are a cerebral hemorrhage and a subarachnoid hemorrhage. The bleeding artery can be caused by head trauma or an aneurysm, which is a blood-filled balloon that leaks blood from a weak spot in the artery wall, and may be caused or aggravated by high-blood pressure. Sudden onset of severe headache with or without vomiting may be the first sign of a hemorrhage. A cerebral hemorrhage occurs when an artery in the brain ruptures and floods the tissue with blood. Finally, a subarachnoid hemorrhage is caused by a blood vessel bursting on the brain's surface. The ruptured vessels fill the space between the brain and the skull with blood, but not the brain itself as in a cerebral hemorrhage.

When a brain hemorrhage occurs, the loss of blood supply means that brain cells can no longer function. Furthermore, the blood puts pressure on the brain tissue and symptoms depend on the amount of pressure put

on the brain tissue. Although hemorrhage-related strokes are more fatal than strokes caused by clots, people who do survive tend to recover better than those who suffer from cerebral thrombosis or cerebral embolism. This is because when the brain cells die, they cannot be repaired. However, when pressure from a hemorrhage is alleviated, the brain can recover.

The way that the stroke affects the individual depends on the type of stroke, the area of the brain that it affects and the severity of the stroke.

A stroke may affect motor skills, speech, behavior and thought patterns, memory and emotions. Stroke survivors may have trouble understanding speech or relaying what they are thinking. This is called aphasia and can affect speaking, reading, writing and listening. Often, the person is paralyzed or weaker on one side of the body. Eyesight on one side of the body can also be affected by a stroke, which causes a person's perception to be off. Finally, stroke survivors may have problems thinking clearly.

Because a stroke can cause permanent brain damage it is important to know the warning signs in order to act quickly.

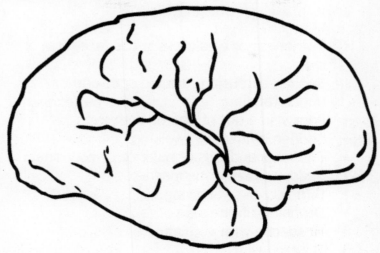

Brain and its blood supply

Signs of a Stroke

- Numbness or weakness in the face, arm or leg.
- Sudden confusion, trouble speaking or understanding.
- Poor vision out of one or both eyes.
- Sudden difficulty in walking.
- Dizziness and loss of balance or coordination.
- Sudden onset of headache.
- Difficulty in swallowing.
- Drooping of one side of face.
- Headache with vomiting.
- Double vision.

The warning signs of a stroke include numbness or weakness in the face, arms or legs, and usually occur on only one side of the body. Other warning signs include sudden confusion, trouble speaking or understanding, and poor vision out of one or both eyes. Also sudden difficulty in walking, dizziness, and loss of balance or coordination are indicators of a stroke. Finally, sudden, severe headaches can signal a stroke. TIAs, which were mentioned above, often do not precede a stroke. Rather, someone who has suffered from a TIA may have a stroke in the future. On average, a TIA last about a minute.

Risk Factors for Having a Stroke

- High blood pressure.
- Diabetes mellitus.
- Carotid artery (neck arteries) disease.
- Atrial fibrillation (irregular heart beat.)
- Smoking.
- Sickle cell anemia.
- High cholesterol.
- Obesity.

Prevention and Maintenance

You must take steps to control weight, keep blood pressure in normal range and monitor cholesterol level to prevent the heart attack or a stoke. One of the best ways to maintain a healthy heart is a good balanced diet and plenty of exercise. A poor diet can lead to obesity, diabetes, high cholesterol and high blood pressure, which are all risk factors that affect the cardiovascular system.

Proteins, carbohydrates and fats are the main component in food. 60 percent of calories should come from complex carbohydrates, 30 percent from fats, with less than 10 percent from saturated fats, and 10 percent from proteins.

Engaging in 45 to 60 minutes of physical activity per day strengthens the heart and helps manage one's weight. Furthermore, not smoking cigarettes and drinking alcohol in moderation will also prevent conditions leading to cardiovascular diseases. By following these simple guidelines, you can keep your heart and the rest of the body healthy and long lasting.

Three Filters

The three filters in the body are the Liver, Lungs and Kidneys. These organs receive blood and purify it by taking out the toxins and nutrients or adding oxygen to the blood for proper body functions. When the blood rich in nutrients from the intestinal area passes through the liver, it absorbs and stores the essential nutrients for the function of the body.

Lungs oxygenate, add oxygen, to the blood and remove carbon dioxide from the circulating blood.

Kidneys control the electrolytes that include sodium, potassium, calcium and chloride among several other items. The kidneys keep the balance of these essential electrolytes for finer tuning of the body functions.

The heart, liver, lungs, and kidneys, to keep you healthy, work together in a dependent harmony. Functions of these organs suffer if blood supply form the heart is reduced for any reason.

Liver

The liver is dark brown in color and triangular in shape; it is located at the right side of the body just under the diaphragm. It is protected partially from the outside by the ribs and the abdominal muscles. It is a unique organ in that it can regenerate itself thus sometimes making partial liver donation a possibility. It has two lobes that are interconnected. The main artery takes blood to the liver and one large vein takes blood out of the liver.

Structure and Function

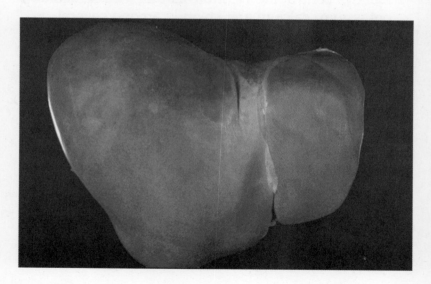

Human Liver

Blood from the stomach and intestine rich in nutrients circulates through the liver. Inside the liver is a fine network of cells and blood vessels that extract the nutrients and break down products of alcohol and drugs. The liver metabolizes a large number of drugs. It also stores carbohydrates. The liver maintains a normal blood sugar level by dealing with carbohydrates. The liver also produces proteins and blood clotting factors. Fats are oxidized in the liver cells. If carbohydrates or sugar is reduced drastically this oxidation produces toxic substances known as ketones.

1500 milliliters of blood pass through the liver in one minute. The liver suffers if its oxygen supply is reduced as in poor circulation in heart failure. The liver metabolizes vitamins specially Vitamin A, D, E and K. Estrogens and steroids are metabolized in the liver and the end products are excreted in the urine. Morphine is metabolized in the liver.

Bile is produced in the liver and excreted into the intestine (gut) via the gall bladder. When there is a blockage in the secretion from the liver to the intestine, the yellow bile results in the yellow appearance of the white part of the eyes and skin known as jaundice. Certain other conditions such as taking sulfa, testosterone, anabolic steroids, gallstones and cancer may also cause jaundice.

Risk Factors

Any infection, injury or substance abuse may result
in the inflammation of the liver cells. This may result
in malfunction of the liver shown by fever, or yellow
color of the eyes and skin. Certain viruses causing
hepatitis can also inflame the liver. Most common
are hepatitis A, hepatitis B and hepatitis C. Hepatitis
C is related to the development of liver cancer if not
treated.

Diseases of the Liver

The liver may be the site of primary or secondary
cancer (cancer spreading from other parts of the
body). Inflammation of the liver results in hepatitis.
Obstruction of the flow of the bile through liver cells
results in the developing of jaundice. Liver cirrhosis
is the result of scarring and failure of liver cells to
function due to alcohol abuse (cirrhosis). This
results in fluid accumulation in the abdomen
(ascites).

Bile and its breakdown products increase in different
conditions of the liver. In obstructive jaundice urine
is dark yellow and stools are pale white in color. In
hemolytic disorder bile salts in the bowel increase
resulting in dark yellow color of stools, and in

infective states urine gets both direct and indirect bilirubin.

Hepatitis A (HAV)

Hepatitis A virus causes an illness with the onset of symptoms that may be delayed for up to 25 days after exposure. Most common symptoms are as follows:

Fever.
Headache.
Weakness.
Nausea.
Abdominal pain.
Vomiting.
Fatigue.
Few days of Jaundice.
Passing dark color urine.
Pale colored stools.

HAV is the most common type of viral hepatitis. It is spread by the oral-fecal route. Infection may occur by household members, sexual contact with an infected person, child day care centers or by international travel.

HIV is preventable by vaccine. Hepatitis A vaccine is easily available. It is important to receive a prophylactic dose before travel to HAV prevalent regions.

Vaccine schedule

Routine vaccination is recommended for high risk group individuals including those traveling to infected areas, men who have sex with men, illegal drug users and those at increased occupational risk of exposure. The vaccine called Havrix should be given by two injections 6-12 months apart and 4 weeks prior to travel to endemic areas.

Hepatitis B (HBV)

Hepatitis B virus causes an illness with slow onset of as long as 75 days after the exposure. The most common symptom of chronic HBV is fatigue. Other symptoms include the following:
Loss of appetite.
Sleep disturbances.
Difficulty concentrating.
Abdominal discomfort.
Nausea.
Vomiting.
Joint pains.
Rash.
Few will develop Jaundice.

Two billion people world wide are infected with HBV and 350 million are chronically infected. It increases the chance of developing cancer of the liver. HBV spreads by exposure to the blood of or through sexual contact with an infected person. Less common sources of infection are by blood transfusion, or by dental treatment by improperly sterilized medical instruments. Infection of newborn may happen from a carrier mother or one with active disease.

Hepatitis Immune Globulin and Hepatitis B vaccine are available for treatment.
Newborns of HBV infected mothers should receive hepatitis B immunoglobulin and HBV vaccine at delivery and follow with remaining vaccines.

Vaccine Schedule

Infants

At birth first dose, remaining doses should be given at 1-2 and 6 months of age.
Vaccine is recommended for all children at 0-18 years of age.

High Risk Group

Hepatitis B vaccine is recommended for persons in the following high risk groups:
Persons coming in contact with blood.
Recipient of blood and blood products.
Hemodialysis patients.

Persons in occupational risk.
Clients and staff of institutions for developmentally disabled.

Household and sexual partners of HBsAg carriers.
Certain international travelers.
Injection drug users.
Persons with HCV infection.

Precautions

Practice safe sex.
Do not take illegal drugs.
Do not share razors, toothbrushes or nail clippers.
Follow universal precautions to avoid direct contact with blood.

Hepatitis C (HCV)

Hepatitis C is a major public health concern. An estimated 4 million people in the United States are infected with HCV. One half of the chronic liver disease is hepatitis C related. 10,000 people die every year due to this infection.

Some of the symptoms may include

Loss of appetite.
Abdominal discomfort.
Nausea.
Vomiting.
Jaundice.
Depression.

Diagnosis

Diagnosis is made by a third generation HCV antibody test.

Are you at risk for Hepatitis C?

You may be at risk if:
You have ever injected illegal drugs, shared needles for tattooing or piercing.
You have ever received treatment for clotting problems with a blood product made before 1987.
You received a blood transfusion or solid organ transplant before 1992.
You were on long term kidney dialysis.
A sex partner has Hepatitis C.
Your mother had HCV before you were born.
You have HIV.

Complications of HCV infection are developing cirrhosis of liver, cancer of liver and liver failure

Liver Transplant is an option but the screening criteria need to be met.

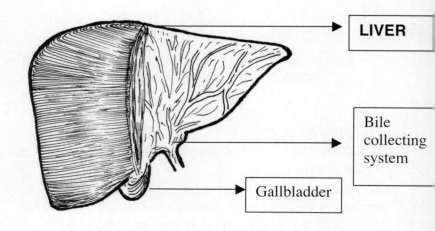

LIVER

Bile
collecting
system

Gallbladder

Maintenance

Protect your liver by avoiding alcohol and toxic
medication and avoiding hepatitis exposure.
Hepatitis vaccine against hepatitis A and B is easily
available and should be used to protect the liver
from further harm. Testing of households is not
necessary unless they had blood exposure. The life
time risk for sexual transmission of HCV in
monogamous couples is less than 1 percent. CDC
does not recommend any changes in sexual practice
in these individuals.

An infant whose mother has hepatitis C should be tested for anti-HCV by 12 months of age. Earlier diagnosis is possible with HCVRNA (PCR) test at 1-2 months of age. An infected mother may breast feed unless nipples are cracked or bleeding.

Treatment, after diagnosis that is made by liver biopsy and blood tests, is available. Type 1 requires 12 months of treatment, type 2 and 3 require only 6 months of treatment. Cure rate is 50-80 percent with combination of pegylated interferon and ribavirin. The cost of therapy is approximately $25,000 for a 48 week course but the treatment has been shown to be cost effective.

Lungs

The lungs come as a pair in the body, one on each side of the heart lying above the diaphragm. They are protected by the ribcage and are connected to the throat through a long tube called the trachea. The trachea is in turn connected to the outside through the mouth and nose. There are two lobes in each lung with an accessory lobe on the right side; these are all interconnected. The diaphragm separates the chest cavity from the abdomen. The hole in the diaphragm is for the food pipe to pass through. If there is any laxity or hernia at this point the usual symptoms are those of heartburn, gas and chest pain. The condition is called reflux, which may happen with or without a hiatus hernia. The respiratory center in the brain controls the breathing movements.

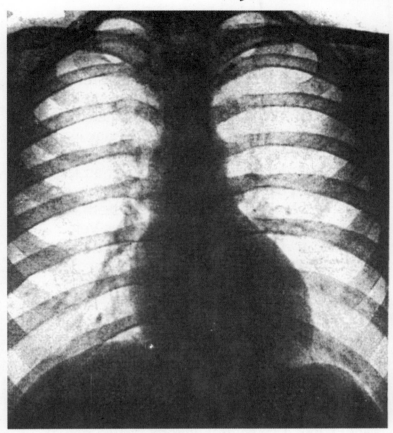

Chest x-ray showing lungs and heart image

Structure and Function

The lungs receive their blood from the right side of the heart and after adding oxygen to it return it to the heart for distribution. The lungs add oxygen to the blood (ventilation) at a rate of 6 liters per minute and during exercise this rate may increase to 100 liters per minute. Lack of blood supply to the lungs results in infarction as in a heart attack, or a blood clot in the blood vessel may result in sudden chest pain, shortness of breath and death if not treated immediately. Blood clots (Deep Vein Thrombosis) may travel from abdominal areas or lower extremities blood vessels. This is more common after abdominal surgery or after prolonged bed rest.

In obesity the ventilation rate is reduced and also in conditions such as head injury, narcotics use and lack of movements of diaphragm. Other conditions that may affect ventilation are lung tumors, pneumonia, asthma and abnormalities of the rib cage. Lungs also control uniform distribution of blood throughout the lungs for oxygenation (perfusion). Perfusion is affected by blood clots (pulmonary embolism). Blood clots in the lung will cause sudden onset of breathing difficulty, chest pain, cough with blood in the sputum, rapid heart beat and pain or swelling in the calf muscles of the leg.

The breathing mechanism consists of breathing in and breathing out controlled by elastic recoil of the chest and function of the brain. Blood gases and lung function can be measured easily to show the status of the lungs (Pulmonary Function Test). Lung transplants are becoming more successful and it is possible to live with just one lung.

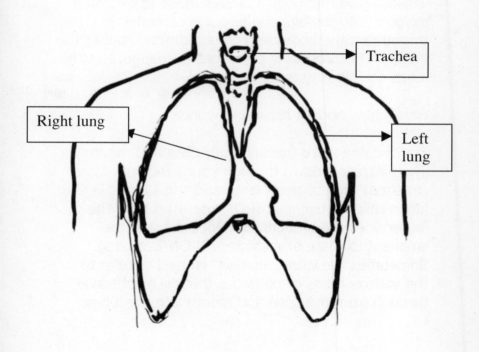

How Do the Lungs Work?

The lungs provide a large surface area for the exchange of oxygen and carbon dioxide between the body and the environment.

Normal lung function. A slice of normal lung looks like a pink sponge—filled with tiny bubbles or holes. Around each bubble is a fine network of tiny blood vessels. These bubbles, surrounded by blood vessels, give the lungs a large surface to exchange oxygen (into the blood where it is carried throughout the body) and carbon dioxide (out of the blood). This process is called gas exchange. Healthy lungs do this very well.

Here's how normal breathing works:

You breathe in air through your nose and mouth. The air travels down through your windpipe (trachea) then through large and small tubes in your lungs called bronchial (BRON-kee-ul) tubes. The larger ones are bronchi (BRONK-eye), and the smaller tubes are bronchioles (BRON-kee-oles). Sometimes the word "airways" is used to refer to the various tubes or passages that air must travel through from the nose and mouth into the lungs.

The airways in your lungs look something like an upside-down tree with many branches.

At the ends of the small bronchial tubes are groups of tiny air sacs called alveoli (al-VEE-uhl-EYE). The air sacs have very thin walls, and small blood vessels called capillaries run in the walls. Oxygen passes from the air sacs into the blood in these small blood vessels. At the same time, carbon dioxide passes from the blood into the air sacs. Carbon dioxide, a normal byproduct of the body's metabolism, must be removed.

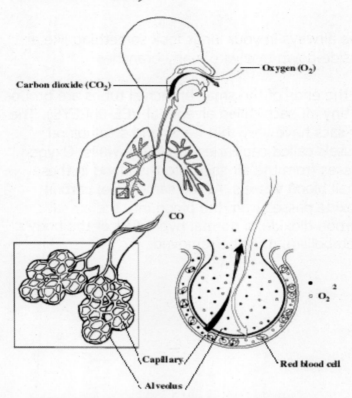

Carbon dioxide (CO_2)

Oxygen (O_2)

CO

O_2^2

Capillary

Red blood cell

Alveolus

Transfer of oxygen of inhaled air into the blood and of waste carbon dioxide of blood into he lungs occur in the alveolus.

The airways and air sacs in the lung are normally elastic-that is, they try to spring back to their original shape after being stretched or filled with air, just the way a new rubber band or balloon would. This elastic quality helps retain the normal structure of the lung and helps to move the air quickly in and out. In chronic obstructive
pulmonary disease, much of the elastic quality is gone, and the airways and air sacs no longer

bounce back to their original shape. This means that the airways collapse, like a floppy hose, and the air sacs tend to stay inflated. The floppy airways obstruct the airflow out of the lungs, leading to an abnormal increase in the lungs' size. In addition, the airways may become inflamed and thickened and mucus-producing cells produce more mucus, further contributing to the difficulty of getting air out of the lungs.

In the type of COPD called emphysema, the walls between the air sacs are destroyed, leading to a few large air sacs, instead of many tiny ones. Then, the lung looks like a sponge with large bubbles or holes in it instead of a sponge with very even tiny holes. These few large air sacs have less surface area than the many tiny ones for the exchange of oxygen and carbon dioxide. *(Source NIH Data)*

Lung ailments may be present as

- Shortness of breath.
- Coughing.
- Wheezing.
- Chest pain.
- Blood in sputum.
- Fever.
- Weakness.
- Difficulty in breathing.

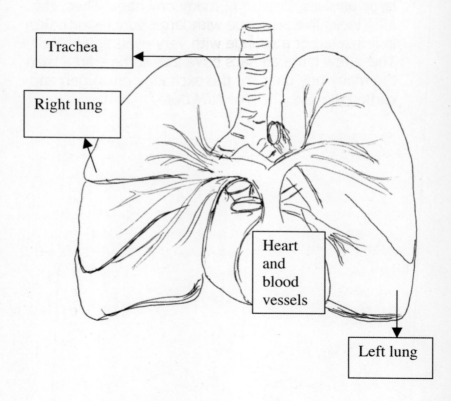

Trachea

Right lung

Heart and blood vessels

Left lung

Diseases of the Lungs

The lungs just as any other part of the body may develop tumors, cancers, puncture wounds, blood clots or infections. As the lungs are involved with breathing first symptoms may appear as difficulty in breathing, coughing, blood in the sputum and chest pain. Cigarette smoking is harmful to the tissue of the lungs.

It causes initially reversible and later irreversible damage to the lungs. Allergies and asthma are due to spasm of the branches of the bronchioles in the wind pipe. This causes cough, audible wheezing and shortness of breath.

Asthma

Asthma is presented as cough, wheezing, and shortness of breath at rest or on exercise, cough at night and after cold air exposure. Diagnosis is made by pulmonary testing (spirometry) that shows airflow obstruction. Several oral medications and inhaled steroids are available to control the symptoms. Triggering factors should be recognized and treated. Flu vaccine should be received annually.

Chronic Obstructive Lung Disease and Emphysema

Chronic obstructive pulmonary disease (COPD) is a lung disease in which the lungs are damaged, making it hard to breathe. In COPD, the airways-the tubes that carry air in and out of your lungs-are partly obstructed, making it difficult to get air in or out. COPD is chronic shortness of breath with obstruction in breathing out. It includes chronic bronchitis and emphysema.

It usually starts as slow shortness of breath that becomes severe over a length of time. A chest X-ray, pulmonary function test and testing blood for gases may help make the diagnosis. Several medical treatments that include bronchodilators are available.

Cigarette smoking is the most common cause of COPD. Most people with COPD are smokers or former smokers. Breathing in other kinds of lung irritants, like pollution, dust, or chemicals over a long period of time may also cause or contribute to COPD.

The airways branch out like an upside-down tree, and at the end of each branch are many small, balloon-like air sacs. In healthy people, each airway is clear and open, the air sacs are small, and both are elastic and springy. When you breathe in, each air sac fills up with air, like a small balloon, and

92

when you breathe out, the balloon deflates and the air goes out.

In COPD, the airways and air sacs lose their shape and become floppy. Less air gets in and less air goes out because:

The airways and air sacs lose their elasticity (like an old rubber band)

The walls between many of the air sacs are destroyed
The walls of the airways become thick and inflamed (swollen)
Cells in the airways make more mucus (sputum) than usual, which tends to clog the airways.

COPD develops slowly, and it may be many years before you notice symptoms like feeling short of breath. Most of the time, COPD is diagnosed in middle-aged or older people.

COPD is a major cause of death and illness throughout the world. It is the 4th leading cause of death in the U.S. and the world.

There is no cure for COPD. The damage to your airways and lungs cannot be reversed, but there are things you can do to feel better and slow the damage to your lungs.

COPD is not contagious-you cannot catch it from someone else.

Lung Cancer

Lung cancer is associated with cigarette smoking and the most common cause of cancer deaths. Diagnosis is by history, x-rays or MRI or biopsy. Prognosis depends on the staging of the disease. Small cell cancer of the lung is the most common. In limited early stages, combination chemotherapy results in a 90% response rate. Median survival of 18 months and cure rate of 5-15% of patients is expected. In non-small cell lung cancer survival rates after treatment have improved very little.

Pneumonia

Pneumonia is a condition where lung tissue is inflamed and infected. Usually a chest x-ray will help make the diagnosis. It may be caused by bacteria, viruses, chemicals or radiation. It is necessary to diagnose and treat pneumonia as early as possible to prevent complications or even death.

Spontaneous Pneumothorax (air outside lungs)

It is described as free air trapped into the pleural space. It usually happens in young people who have congenital abnormality in their lung tissue or in older people who have emphysema or pulmonary fibrosis.

Pneumothorax is presented with shortness of breath and chest pain. There are two layers of pleura covering the surface of each lung. Air enters from the lung tissue and is not due to injury or trauma. It is sometimes self limiting and improves by itself. Other treatments available are insertion of a chest tube under a seal and draining the air out of the pleural space.

Risk Factors

Breathing fresh air is necessary for the function of lungs, which is to add oxygen to the blood. If lung capacity is reduced then the individual does not get enough oxygen in the system resulting in fatigue, inability to sleep or breathe. Smoking cigarettes causes lung damage and produces cough. This may result in development of cancer.

Radiation treatment and exposure result in scarring and reduced functional capacity of the lungs. This causes shortness of breath and persisting cough. Infections such as pneumonia may result in temporary or permanent damage to the lung tissue and reduce its function to exchange gases.

In conditions such as asthma, there is spasm of the bronchioles, the air tubes in the lung, resulting in a wheezing, cough and difficulty in breathing.

Chronic respiratory diseases and emphysema also interfere with the proper function of the lungs. Environmental exposure such as smoke and fumes, pollens and other obnoxious toxins cause irritation to the lung tissue.

Maintenance

Prevention of pneumonia is achievable by getting protection with influenza vaccine and pneumonia vaccine.

Pneumonia vaccine

Pneumococcal vaccination should be considered for high risk population. Usually one shot is necessary; a second shot is recommended for people age 65 and older who received their first dose when they were under 65 and if 5 or more years have passed since the last dose.

Influenza vaccine protects against flu virus and should be taken every year.

Protect your lungs by avoiding breathing polluted air. Air contaminated with fumes, smoke, dust or chemicals may damage the inner lining of the airways and lung tissue. The inner lining of the air passages such as nose, mouth, throat, and windpipe is lined with filaments or cilia and supplied with an increased amount of blood. This cools the inhaled air and prevents any foreign particles from entering the lungs. The wind pipe (trachea) is located in the middle of the throat. If it is pushed to one side, its position usually indicates a growth pushing the windpipe to one side.

The windpipe divides in to two branches, the right and the left bronchus. The right branch is straighter than the left. A foreign body may lodge easily in the right side of the bronchus. Allergic reactions or spasms of the air tubes may result in difficulty in breathing and an audible wheezing noise as seen in asthma. Each lung is covered with a sheath of thin layer called pleura. If there is a puncture wound to the chest, air can enter into the pleura causing collapse of the lung, a condition called pneumothorax (air in the chest outside the lungs).

Kidneys

The kidneys are in a pair and are located on each side of the mid spine in the body, well cushioned and connected to the main blood supply (aorta) in the abdomen. The blood supply comes directly from the aorta by the renal arteries and the blood is drained back via inferior vena cava. One quarter of the heart's output flows through the kidneys every minute, that is 1200 milliliters/minute (approximately 5 cups per minute).

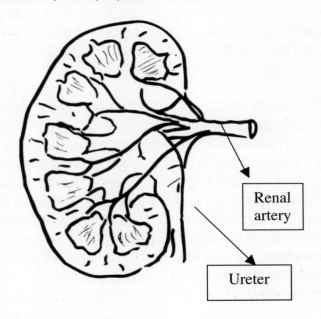

Renal artery

Ureter

Blood supply of the kidney

Structure and Function

The blood is filtered in the kidneys by a very fine network of tubes. A lot happens at these tubes as blood flows through them, adding and excreting electrolytes and nutrients. The kidneys excrete water, glucose, creatinine, ammonia, sodium, potassium, calcium, magnesium, chloride, phosphate, sulphate, proteins, urea and uric acid. The kidneys also absorb certain nutrients and electrolytes as blood passes through the kidney tubules. Other than excreting toxic materials the kidneys regulate the acid base balance of the body.

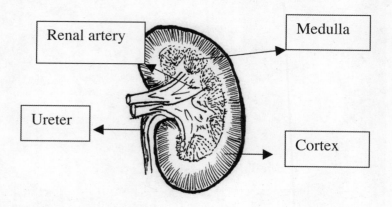

The kidneys maintain heart output by controlling pressure in the arteries (blood vessels). Kidney function also controls sodium (salt) excretion. In conditions that interfere with the blood flow in the kidneys, salt is retained causing water to accumulate in the body. This water retention can cause shortness of breath, fluid in the lungs or swelling of the ankles.

Exercise increases the heart rate and circulation through the kidneys allowing more blood to go through the filtration process. Early sign of pump failure (heart
failure) is decreased circulation and less production of urine.

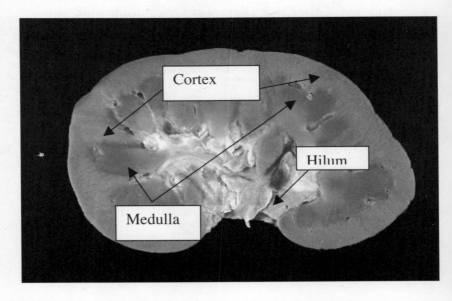

Cortex

Hilum

Medulla

The kidney consists of an outer part, the cortex and an inner part, called medulla. There is one square meter of tubes inside one million capsules measuring approximately 0.2mm in diameter in both kidneys. Each kidney via a tube called the ureter excretes waste. Each side ureter drains urine into the bladder where it is stored until it is emptied. The ureter is attached on the one side to the hilum of the kidney and on the other side to the bladder.

Urine production

Urine production varies with the intake of fluids, kidney conditions, concurrent illness, exercise, body temperature and outside temperature. Daily output of urine varies between 1000 to 1500 milliliters (5-6 cups a day). Urine is normally free of glucose and proteins (albumin) except in diabetes and after exercise. The yellow color of urine is due to the pigment urochrome. The color becomes darker in dehydration, fever and after exercise. Urea breakdown to ammonia in the urine is responsible for the odor in urine.

Common Problems and Complications

Blood in the urine

Hematuria or blood in the urine could be variable in nature from microscopic (not visible by the naked eye) or frank hematuria where red color urine is passed. There are several causes of having blood in the urine. Kidney tumors or infections may produce blood in the urine. Other causes include, injuries, blood disorders, taking blood thinners such as coumadin, kidney stones and few other less common conditions. Certain drugs also cause dark colored urine. These include sulfa, methyldopa, metronidazole pyridium and levodopa.

Urinary tract infection

Urinary tract infection may involve kidneys and produce fever, chills, dark color urine, frequency of urination and difficulty in emptying the bladder. Kidney failure results after suffering an acute illness or in chronic illness such as diabetes. This results in accumulation of toxic substances in the blood and may need kidney dialysis or kidney transplant.

Normal health can be maintained with one kidney as seen in live donor situations.

Test

Kidney function may be measured by a blood test indicating levels of creatinine and urea.

When there is a problem with the kidney

It may cause

- Pain in the back or abdomen.
- Fever and chills.
- Frequency of urination.
- Burning sensation when passing urine.
- Inability to pass urine.
- Blood in the urine.
- Weakness.
- Anemia.
- High blood pressure.
- Fluid retention.

Common Diseases

Pyelonephritis.
Nephritis.
Kidney Stone.
Kidney Enlargement (Hydronephrosis).
Kidney (Renal) Failure.
Kidney tumors and cysts.

Risk Factors

Kidneys are at risk of impaired function if they are under any stress. Kidneys play a major role in controlling and maintaining blood pressure. Any infection in the urinary tract or obstruction such as an enlarged prostate gland in males and kidney stones may lead to retention of urine or risk of increasing infection.

Intravenous dyes (contrast material injected prior to certain procedures) as used in CAT scan and x-rays may over time damage kidney function. Kidney function is assessed by a blood test called creatinine and urinary output.

Renal failure results in changes in blood pressure, weakness due to related anemia, swelling of ankles and fluid retention.

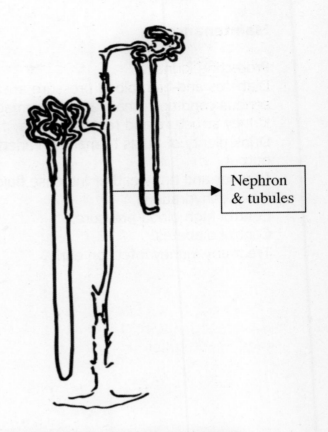

Nephron & tubules

Nephron and collecting tubules inside the kidney

Maintenance

Protecting kidneys:
Diabetes and high blood pressure are the two most serious conditions that result in damage to the kidney structure and result in kidney failure.
Drink plenty of fluids to maintain adequate urine output.
In fever and hot weather increase fluid intake to avoid dehydration.
Control high blood pressure.
Control diabetes.
Treat any kidney infection early.

Rule of Three

- Eat three times a day.
- Exercise three times a week.
- Walk at least three miles at a stretch.

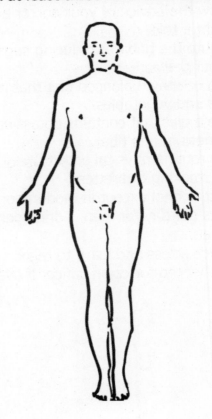

Lifestyle Changes

You can help yourself to better manage your own health.

- Follow the advice of your doctor and lose weight if told.
- Get into the habit of reducing sugar and salt in your diet.
- Eat a healthy, balanced diet that includes fruits and vegetables.
- Have a diet that contains potassium, calcium, magnesium and fiber.
- Start routine physical activity.
- Quit smoking cigarettes.
- Avoid alcohol except in moderation. 1-2 drinks per day for men, I drink per day for women.
- Reduce stress and learn to relax.
- Get checked for colon cancer if over age 50.

Ayaz M. Samadani M.D.

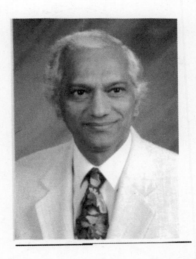

Ayaz M. Samadani M.D., DCH. (London), DTM&H.
(Liverpool)

Chair Public Health Council,
The Department of Public Health and Family
Services of
the State of Wisconsin.

Member International Health Advisory Committee,
University of Wisconsin Medical School, Madison,
Wisconsin, U.S.A.

Filter
Lungs
Pump
Heart
Filter
Liver
Filter
Kidneys

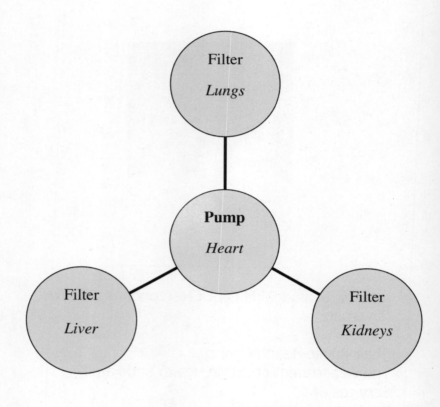

Three Filters and a Pump